Wheels of Change

How Complex Rehab Technology was Born, Evolved, and
Fosters the Independence of Americans with Disabilities

Mark E. Smith

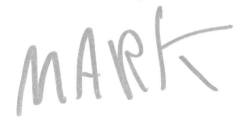

Wheels of Change
How Complex Rehab Technology was Born, Evolved, and Fosters the
Independence of Americans with Disabilities

Cover photo by Emily C. Smith, www.emilyslens.com

ISBN-13: 978-1492200710
ISBN-10:1492200719

Other Books by Mark E. Smith

Making the Most of It: The 11 Keys to Mastering Disability and Life

Too Fast: Selected True Tales from the Madman of WheelchairJunkie.com

Growing Up With Cerebral Palsy: A Remarkable Story by San Francisco's Impossible Dream Kid

To my daughter, Emily – my truest inspiration.

Contents

Part Two: Complex Rehab, the Bold New World

Part Three: Complex Rehab, the Mainstream

Part Four: CMS Intervention and Congressional Legislation

Afterword

Foreword
By Don Clayback

For the past four years, I've had the honor of serving as Executive Director of NCART, the National Coalition for Assistive and Rehab Technology. NCART is a national organization of complex rehab technology providers and manufacturers focused on protecting access (i.e. coverage and payment) for people with disabilities and chronic medical conditions. I came into the industry in 1985 and have witnessed and participated in many of the changes over these years. I've spent time as a complex rehab technology specialist, ran a complex rehab technology company, worked as an industry consultant, and now advocate to promote and protect access. It's safe to say complex rehab technology is in my blood.

Now, *complex rehab technology* – or *CRT* as we affectionately call it – is quite a mouthful. In plain English, I usually translate it as, "specialized wheelchairs, seating systems, and other adaptive equipment used by people with disabilities." The term *complex rehab technology* is technical and formal; but, unfortunately, that's what's called for in the nomenclature of policy makers and funding organizations. However, the essence of CRT means so much more to so many people. As Mark states in his first chapter, "It's a very formal term for a very personal subject." This book provides the foundation and real life stories that support that statement.

How appropriate it is that Mark writes about the history and evolution of CRT. He not only has an inspiring personal life story as a CRT user, but he is a tireless advocate and has been carrying the CRT message far and wide his whole adult life. If someone was looking for an excellent example of what a person with a disability can do given the right technology, they need go no further than the successful website Mark created at www.wheelchairjunkie.com. His personal story, writings, and professional career provide amazing testimony to individual commitment, determination, and the important role that CRT can play in someone's life.

Forty plus years of history is a lot to cover, but that's just what this book does. It traces the evolution of CRT in an informative and comfortable style. It's encouraging to read how advancements in technology and improvements in the service delivery process truly improved the quality of life for millions of people with disabilities. Mark acknowledges that he could not include all of the dedicated organizations and individuals that played a part in getting CRT to where it is today. But, he does an excellent job of providing highlights and insights that will be of interest to anyone that uses, prescribes, provides, or manufactures CRT.

Our country has done a lot to help people with disabilities. The *Americans with Disabilities Act* and the subsequent investment of billions of dollars to provide community access through ramps, curb cuts, public transportation, building accessibility, and other improvements are good examples. However, the reality is that without access to the right mobility and seating (i.e., complex rehab technology) these improvements do nothing for a person with a disability who relies on a wheelchair to get around and carry on the activities of daily life. For hundreds of thousands of people, the right wheelchair is the starting point of access – that's why the technological advancements in CRT are so important and empowering. The principle extends to all CRT items, including gait trainers, standers, and other specialized adaptive equipment.

This underscores the necessity of protecting access to CRT through adequate coverage and funding. Unfortunately, today's pressures to reduce healthcare costs can take the form of indiscriminate cuts, and this small category of specialized products is very vulnerable. The starting point in protecting CRT access is to create a much higher awareness and understanding of what CRT is all about: who uses it, how it's provided, and the medical, social, and economic benefits it brings. Needing particular emphasis is the significant labor and expertise that is required to get people the right CRT equipment initially, and then to support its use with service and repairs. We need to be better understood and accepted by federal, state, and private healthcare policy makers and funding entities. This is an effort that all CRT stakeholders must play an active part in. Helpful information can be found at www.access2crt.org.

This book takes you through the evolution of CRT, from its humble start to its current day status. Mark does a great job highlighting key events that have taken place from both the perspective of an industry observer and a CRT consumer. I'm confident anyone with a connection to or interest in complex rehab technology will enjoy reading this book and gain important details and insight about the history of CRT and, most importantly, the roles it plays in liberating those with disabilities.

Don Clayback

Executive Director, NCART

September 2013

Author's Note

The professional field now known as *complex rehab technology*, as with all movements that truly contribute positive change to society and culture, wasn't born of a single person. Rather, countless practitioners, inventors, researchers, manufacturers, providers, and those with disabilities have all equally, greatly contributed to its genesis and evolution. And, every person, technology, and service in this field deserves exceptional recognition in contributing to the remarkable impact made toward liberating the lives of those with disabilities.

In this book you will read the awe-inspiring stories of those who've made significant contributions toward complex rehab technology, revealing a never-before-documented story of the industry with fascinating personalities at the helm. Some names you'll learn, some names you'll recognize, and some names were, by the limited nature of print, left out. Yet, all should be acknowledged. For every Gerry Dickerson there's an Elaine Trefler, and for every LaBac tilt system there's a Falcon. The list goes on and on, with each person, product, and service no less important than those compiled within the binding of this book.

Likewise, complex rehab technology has evolved in different ways, at different times, in different countries. This book's intent isn't to overlook the global markets, but to focus specifically on the United States, where the lack of globalization and communication technologies of the 1970s and 1980s didn't allow the global exchanges that we have today toward products, practices, regulations, and services.

Indeed, although it's impossible to note everyone who's impacted complex rehab, the innovators, ground-breaking products, and pivotal moments in this text were cross-referenced as emblematic of the snapshots in time when they occurred. In this way, it's my intention that you, the reader, will not only find yourself engaged by the remarkable anecdotes within, but also not forget about the countless individuals not mentioned who likewise profoundly affected not just the complex rehab industry, but every individual with a disability who his or her work touched

Acknowledgments

At the center of complex rehab technology is the human heart. In writing the body of this work that truth was more evident than ever in the generosity, inspiration, and passion that so many contributed to this book through their words, wisdom, and astounding contributions to the most noble of fields, complex rehab technology.

In alphabetical order, I wish to thank Marty Ball, Mike Ballard, Paul Bergantino, Adrienne Falk Bergen, Mary Wilson Boegel, Don Clayback, Gerry Dickerson, James Doty, Gary Gilberti, Marilyn Hamilton, Mark Kettler, Paul Komishock, Michele Leahy, Scott Meuser, Mal Mixon, Jim Mulhern, Joyce Murland, Greg Peek, Hymie Pogir, Dennis Sharpe, Michael Silverman, Haley Taffera, Mark Wels, Jim Wyman, Andrew Yarborough, and countless others who supported this project along the way.

Introduction

Complex rehab technology is a very formal term for a very personal subject – one that's improved the lives of countless Americans with disabilities over approximately the past forty years, fostering the health and freedom needed to pursue education, career, family, and community. I am one of those individuals.

When I was five years old, with severe cerebral palsy, I had no independence and was presumably destined for institutionalization. Sure, I had a manual wheelchair, but based on virtually no coordination or balance, not only couldn't I move my manual wheelchair an inch, but if I was on the floor, with a toy across the room, it might as well have been across an ocean, impossible for me to obtain.

However, one day in physical therapy during the summer of 1976, my therapist had the insight to let me try a power wheelchair. Back then, power wheelchairs were little more than manual wheelchairs with motors and a joystick, but they still allowed those with the severest of disabilities to move about independently.

I remember the therapist sitting me in the power wheelchair, my body twisted like a pretzel, spasmodic beyond control. I swear she must have used every belt and strap that she could find just to anchor me to the seat. Then, using every ounce of coordination that I had, I pushed the joystick, gliding across the room. To me, it was a magic carpet, giving me something I'd never known: the feeling of liberation.

I don't know if you've ever experienced or imagined what it's like to be physically trapped in your own body, but the closest simile that I can make is that it's like being in the cruelest of prisons with no hope of ever being freed. Yet, using that power wheelchair, even for those few moments that day, showed me that there was hope that through the right clinicians and technology, my life could have potential, I could be freed from my prison.

Indeed, I eventually got my own power wheelchair, and it set my life in motion, where I became one of the first severely physically disabled students mainstreamed into California's public school system. I graduated high school, went on to college, established a career, and raised a family. Yet, here's what fascinated me over all of those decades as one thriving with a severe disability. Yes, my tenacity has had a lot to do with my successes; however, so has complex rehab technology and the innovators behind it. I dare say that my life and those of my generation's lives paralleled the development of complex rehab technology beyond coincidence. The better the technology and applications, the greater our independence and opportunities. I've been fascinated by how the independent living movement, including the *Americans with Disabilities Act of 1990*, was fueled by complex rehab technology – as are millions of lives today – and there's a fascinating story therein, from circa 1974 to the present.

All of this leads to the fundamental question of, *What is*

complex rehab technology? In practical terms, it's the adaptation and customization of the wheelchair and seating to the individual. That sounds simple enough, but let me give you a glimpse of how profound that truly is. For a quadriplegic, it's a power wheelchair steered by puffs of breath, with power tilt seating to prevent pressure sores, allowing him or her to be liberated from a life spent in a hospital bed. For a paraplegic, it's an individually-fit ultralight manual wheelchair better suited for independent living, including going to work each day. And, for one with any number of permanent, severe physical disabilities, it's the individualized mobility technology that provides them the liberation to achieve a level of health and quality of life that everyone deserves.

It's the larger role of complex rehab technology that has tremendous positive social impact. When we provide someone the individualized mobility and positioning products needed to pursue education, career, family, and community – that is, the mobility and positioning needed to fully integrate one with a disability into society – we not only increase that person's quality of life, but actually increase his or her contribution to society. We know that the right mobility technology allows one with a severe disability to pursue education, exponentially increasing his or her employment and income levels. Likewise, we know that the right mobility technology dramatically improves a person's health, reducing medical costs. When combined, these factors demonstrate the intrinsic personal and social value to complex rehab technology. It takes an individual from being caught in the governmental financial system, to being self-supporting, paying into the system. Therefore, there's both a quality of life and socio-economic return on complex rehab technology that's quantifiable.

This isn't a book about clinical theory or just feel-good stories. It's about real people, with real vision, where the rubber hit the road, and seemingly ordinary men and women who did extraordinary acts of compassionate, insightful innovation to better the lives of those with disabilities. Like all great evolution-of-an-industry stories, the one of complex rehab technology starts in a garage. Through twists and turns along the way, it ultimately becomes a science-based part of the healthcare community serving countless Americans – and the first person anecdotes by those who were there are both fascinating and awe-inspiring. In whole, it's the story of how, over approximately forty years, the convergence of social awareness, physical need, and innovation created not just technology, but a cultural shift in how those with disabilities are viewed and what they can achieve.

Part One

Where Complex Rehab Technology was Born

When There Was Only Confinement....

In early 1972, Geraldo Rivera, then an investigative reporter for WABC-TV in New York, did a Peabody Award-winning expose' titled *Willowbrook: The Last Disgrace.* What Rivera showed New Yorkers, and ultimately the country, were the horrors occurring to those with physical disabilities behind the doors of Staten Island's Willowbrook State School, an institution housing 6,000 children with disabilities at its peak. Abuse of all forms was rampant within the institution, children with disabilities locked away from society, with no safety net. The nation soon became outraged, and Willowbrook – and other institutions like it – was ultimately cleaned up and closed down.

Still, for all with severe disabilities in the early 1970s and the preceding decades, life was bleak, even in the best of circumstances.

"I remember the world being such an isolated, cold place," recalls Andrew Yarborough, born in 1962, with osteogenesis imperfecta (commonly known as "brittle bones" disease). "Not only were those of us with physical disabilities known as 'invalids' and sent to special schools, but there was no such thing as accessibility. And, the wheelchair of the day was a steel, manual, one-size-fits-all hospital-type. For me, the wheelchairs weren't just restrictive, but they were dangerous. A lack of positioning in the seating or outdoor capabilities kept most of us home-bound. It really was about *confinement* back then."

In fact, prior to the mid-1970s, the wheelchair in its form hadn't changed since it went from wicker to steel in 1933, an invention by Herbert A. Everest and H.C. Jennings that became the industry standard. Weighing in at over 50 pounds, it was, as Yarborough describes, a "hospital" wheelchair, with a simple sling upholstery seat, non-adaptable frame, and skinny solid tires for indoor use only.

Yarborough's experience wasn't unique. For Joyce Murland, born in 1937, her recollections of life growing up with disability prior to modern technological and social advances are telling.

"There simply weren't wheelchairs around when I was growing up," explains Murland, who's a C1-C2 quadriplegic since birth due a doctor incorrectly using forceps to remove her from the womb. "I remember a single gentleman who had an old wheelchair-trike kind of device that he'd used to get up and down the road, and people were fascinated by it. But, that was the only wheelchair that I ever saw."

Murland had to resort to scooting on her belly for mobility, and didn't start school till age seven. "The only educational opportunities for me as a very young child were institutionalization," shares Murland, "so my parents kept me home as long as they could."

Eventually, Murland attended a local school where her only means of mobility was being carried by others. "It was a multi-story school like they all were back then and I remember not only feeling undignified as I was carried around, but I was truly scared being carried up and down the stairs," she shares.

Beyond the harsh physical realities, Murland painfully recalls the social stigmas placed upon her. "The teachers thought that they might somehow catch my disease, even though I didn't have one. Looking back, life for me was so undignified based on the ignorance of others. But, as a child with a disability in those days, I just didn't know any different, so I just went through it the best that I could."

For Jim Wyman, born with cerebral palsy quadriplegia in 1938, he, too, struggled with the lack of technology and faced social stigmas. "Early on, I used a tricycle to scoot around, but by age 7, I attended school in a wagon," explained Wyman, who didn't get his first wheelchair until the 1950s. "I think my dad ordered it from the Sears catalog, but it kept breaking, constantly needing fixing."

Wyman went to college for engineering, and recalls isolation through all of school. "I just never had friends," he recalls. "I just learned to be alone. It's just how it was."

In 1970, Wyman purchased among the first power "production" wheelchairs in the U.S. "It was basically a motorized manual wheelchair that was very limited," shares Wyman. "You

3

had no speed control over it. The joystick was really just an on-off switch with no speed variation. It was go-and-stop. And, there were no brakes. If you wanted to stop, you put it in reverse and hoped for the best."

Wyman further recognized the overall lack of technology and services. "There was no such thing as a 'wheelchair specialist' or even therapists who knew anything about mobility technology or seating and positioning," he explains. "If you needed a solution, you either made it yourself or did without."

For me and others in the early 1970s and proceeding decades, Wyman's experience was all of our experiences with severe disability and mobility technology. I was unable to position myself on a wheelchair's sling upholstery, so my neighbor built me a wedge out of plywood, upholstered it, and it was my first positioning product. All of my peers similarly had wheelchairs that were garage-assembled with wood and sheet metal, all adapting the one-size-fits-all generic wheelchair to each of our specific, individual needs the best that we could.

Still, there was only so much that could be done with the existing technology, where professional practice was non-existent. Power wheelchairs were truly built for indoor use only, so we had little ability to go outdoors. There was no such technology as seating and positioning products, so poor posture and pressure sores were commonplace. And, there were no clinical services. The culmination of these realities left most with disabilities home-bound at best, institutionalized at worst.

Indeed, it was a time when those of us with disabilities weren't just labeled "invalids," we were seen as *invalid* by most of society.

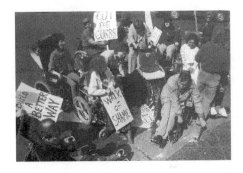

1970s Disability Rights Rally

For the First Time, the Wheelchair was Built for the Individual....

By the mid 1970s, the population of wheelchair users continued increasing – from permanently-wounded veterans of the Vietnam war to polio survivors – and "rehabilitation clinics" were on the rise, serving as a catalyst toward not only meeting the medical needs of those with disabilities, but also teaching independent living skills, right down to sports and recreation.

Leading the way was Rancho Los Amigos National Rehabilitation Center in Downey, California, a cutting-edge facility till this day. At Rancho Los Amigos, circa 1975, worked recreational therapist and paraplegic, Jeff Minnebraker. As a pioneer in wheelchair sports, Minnebraker recognized that mobility was about both everyday independence and optimal performance. And, Minnebraker wanted to improve both, better integrating the individual with his or her wheelchair. Minnebraker's concept was simple but revolutionary: rather than place individuals in one-size-fits-all manual wheelchairs that were a contradiction to ergonomic propulsion, Minnebraker sought to fit and build a manual wheelchair around the individual. The result was using materials like ultralight aluminum instead of stainless steel; reshaping the wheelchair so that it followed the lines of the user's body instead of simply resembling a kitchen chair form; and, making the frame rigid instead of folding, for increased propulsion efficiency.

Soon, in his garage, Minnebraker welded up the first

ultralight wheelchair, one fit to his body, disability, and lifestyle needs. It changed *everything* about how wheelchairs interfaced with users from that moment on, defining a vision, practice, and technology that we now call the genre of *complex rehab.*

For Minnebraker, having a wheelchair that fit his personal needs was life-changing, realizing that a wheelchair could be an extension of his body. In his role at Rancho Los Amigos and within the emerging wheelchair sports community, Minnebraker shared his vision, with his garage becoming a homegrown manufacturing facility, making custom wheelchairs for friends and patients.

As word spread, the legendary liberation of Minnebraker's wheelchairs grew – sleeker, stronger, faster – and an official company was born, Quadra. However, the old-school wheelchair industry wasn't yet buying into the concept of *custom mobility*, as an Everest & Jennings' (the industry leader at the time) executive explained that custom wheelchairs might only serve one percent of the population.

Yet, for Quadra and its growing team, having moved into a manufacturing facility, that supposedly only one percent was exploding. Pioneer track and road racer, Marty Ball, who uses a wheelchair due to polio, worked as a provider at Mobility Unlimited in New York at the time, and was among the first to promote this revolutionary new concept within the clinician community.

"I did in-services with the Quadra, and therapists

immediately understood it," explains Ball. "I showed them the ergonomic shape, ultralight weight, and adjustability – and they got it. For the first time, they realized that a wheelchair could be truly fit and customized to the client."

Indeed, if there was a cataclysmic explosion that ignited the philosophy of complex rehab technology, it occurred in Jeff Minnebraker's garage, with Quadra as Ground Zero. A wave was set in motion that would soon go from revolutionary to evolutionary....

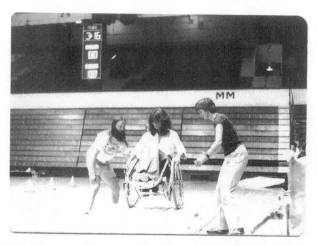

Mary Wilson Boegel Practicing a Wheelie in a Quadra Serial #2 Production Model

A "Quickie" Move Sets the Industry Ablaze....

Among those to admire the Quadra design philosophy was Marilyn Hamilton, paralyzed to T-12 in a hang gliding accident in 1978. Her two hang gliding partners, Jim Okamoto and Don Helman, built hang gliders in a shed on Helman's father's property, and they, along with Hamilton, saw the perfect mix of technical savvy and vision to evolve the ultralight wheelchair design, not just in form, but philosophy. However, none had true business experience, with Okamoto working at a motorcycle shop, Helman a UPS driver, and Hamilton helping her uncle in agriculture. Yet, they knew what they wished to accomplish.

"The goal was pretty simple," recalls Hamilton, now retired from the mobility industry. "We not only wanted to create better mobility and movement, but actually improve people's lives with wheelchairs, making them feel better about themselves with eye-catching style."

In 1979, Motion Designs, Inc. (MDI) was born in the shed on the Helman property. With passion and zeal, Hamilton stormed the country with the refined Quickie ultralight wheelchair, aptly named by Helman after an innovative hang glider wing. Hamilton's marketing savvy, along with Okamoto and Helman's design talents, quickly garnered the attention of providers and consumers. As a Wharton Business School case study on Motion Designs noted, "From the beginning, MDI positioned itself as a focused differentiator. MDI targeted the rehab market and sought to enhance the lives of users, refuting the idea that they were

9

invalids. Like Hamilton, most of MDI's customers had been active before experiencing spinal cord injuries or degenerative diseases. Full-time Quickie users were typically between the ages of 18 and 30 and tended to be people who wanted to remain independent and active."

While MDI's initial success, much like Quadra's, centered around the active and wheelchair sports communities, Hamilton recognized that the same technological advances could be applied toward a much broader demographic, namely those with more severe disabilities. In an industry first, MDI invented the ultralight folding frame, and then began adding option like supportive armrests, flip-up foot plates, high-mount brakes, and an innovation called "hill holders," allowing those with limited strength to push up hills without rolling backward. Projection hand rims were an option for quadriplegics with limited grip, and rear anti-tip wheels were added for those with limited balance.

Indeed, the MDI trio started where Quadra left off, and evolved ultralight wheelchair technology toward meeting the custom mobility needs of those with more severe disabilities through a level of modularity and adaptability that the industry had never known.

MDI's sales continued skyrocketing, averaging over 100 percent annual sales growth, as it created an expanded complex rehab technology market. Dick H. Chandler, C.E.O. of Sunrise Medical, a medical device manufacturer that ultimately purchased MDI, observed at the time, "Motion Designs has been the greatest success story in the rehab industry over the past four years. Their market share exceeds 50 percent in the fastest-growing and highest-margin product segment."

"My interest was not from a business perspective. Not at all. It was totally selfish. I wanted to look nicer and have more function, more mobility, more freedom, more movement," Hamilton shared in a *New Mobility* magazine profile.

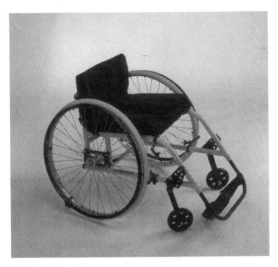

MDI's Quickie

In the First Person: Doug's Story

I was in the sixth grade, which would have been 1982, and dodgeball was popular at my school. I'd used a typical, steel manual wheelchair my whole life. We called them "depot" chairs because they came from the depot closet at the therapy center. It's all I knew, and as an above-the-knee amputee from birth, I wore prosthetic legs simply for aesthetics, and struggled to push my heavy, oversized wheelchair around school, watching from the sidelines as others played dodgeball.

I remember being at Gemco, which was like a Target or Walmart, and I ran into a couple who used wheelchairs. But, unlike my boxy, chrome depot chair, theirs were sleek, colorful, and looked super light. One was labeled Quickie and the other, Quadra. I was fascinated, and the couple showed me all of the adjustability and how easy the chairs were to push. They glided down the store aisle seemingly ten times easier than my chair. I showed my mom and she was fascinated, too.

My father was a successful engineer, and so when my mother and I later brought home brochures from the DME, Dad was likewise intrigued. The ultralight designs could definitely make my life easier and more independent. My parents filed a claim with our insurance and, fortunately, a Quadra was approved.

On the day my Quadra was delivered, I was fitted for it at the therapy center. I remember the first thing I noticed was that it actually fit me and was comfortable. From the first push, I was astounded by how easy it was to propel. I could push myself farther and faster than I ever imagined. I couldn't wait to go to school in my new chair and play dodgeball.

People don't always realize how important the right wheelchair is. But, I can tell you through the eyes of a once sixth grader, who just wanted to play dodgeball with all of the other kids, that the right wheelchair changes your life.

Complex Rehab Technology Powers Up....

With the ultralight manual wheelchair market all the rage in a burgeoning complex rehab segment, Mal Mixon, CEO of the then up-and-coming Ohio-based wheelchair manufacturer, Invacare, saw the next evolution: power wheelchairs.

"When I fully took the reins of Invacare in 1980, the Goliath power chair maker was Everest & Jennings," recalls Mixon. "We knew we could do it better, but had to get our foot in the door."

Mixon saw the impact that the Quickie philosophy had on the market, and was inspired to similarly raise the bar in power mobility.

"I was so impressed by what Motion Designs was doing in manuals that we talked about buying them early on," notes Mixon. "However, Marilyn [Hamilton] and I were never able to reach a deal. But, we knew we could do power really well, regardless."

Mixon put a small team on creating Invacare's own ultralight manual wheelchair line, but focused mainly on revolutionizing complex rehab power, inspired by a personal connection.

"J.B. Richey, who was the inventor behind Invacare's majority of products, was friends with legendary disability rights advocate, Evan Kemp," shares Mixon. "Evan was an attorney and knew all of the boys on Capitol Hill, going on to help legislate the ADA. I remember J.B. and me being on the town with Evan, and his chair died, so we struggled to get him and the chair home. We knew we could make a better power chair. So, J.B. went to work...."

The result was that by 1983, Invacare launched its power chair creation, the Rolls Arrow, complete with industry-leading side shrouding and decal graphics featuring an arrow-type design – sleek and stylish.

"I got in the competitor's chair, rolled down a hill, and the darn thing wouldn't stop, it had no brakes!" Mixon recollects with a chuckle. "I thought, 'Man, how can people with disabilities use a power chair with no brakes?' So, we put brakes on ours, with J.B. coming up with regenerative braking. From there, we just kept improving over the competitor's design till we had the best at that time."

Invacare's Rolls Arrow also introduced the first solid-state, programmable electronics. "We listened to the market, and understood that those with disabilities were diverse," says Mixon. "So, we knew we had to invent electronics and steering that could be tailored to the person."

Hymie Pogir, who signed on with Mixon as a salesman six months after Mixon purchased the then-ailing wheelchair company in 1978, notes of Mixon's vision in the early 1980s, "Mal always understood complex rehab – that was his thing – long before others did. He was always passionate about it."

Invacare's power chair, infused with the first generation of complex rehab technology for those with severe disabilities, immediately began making waves as the most user-centric model on the market and established Invacare as a market force.

With both the manual and power wheelchair markets focused on complex rehab "bases," there was an area still overlooked, but soon to come into the mix: seating and positioning....

An Idea Pulled out of Thin Air....

The fact is, the human body didn't evolve over thousands of years to reside in a seated position, concentrating approximately 75 percent of one's weight on the thin tissue of the buttocks. For full-time wheelchair users, ischemic ulcers and pressure sores (commonly called bed sores), have always been a costly, even deadly issue. And, prior to the 1970s, the risks were at record highs, with wheelchair users sitting on nothing more than vinyl or canvas sling upholstery. As a result, 80 percent of full-time wheelchair users experienced ischemic ulcers and pressure sores.

Circa 1970, Robert H. Graebe was an electrical engineer, working on a project at a hospital. While at the hospital, Graebe noticed the alarming number of pressure sore cases. With no formal training of anatomy, physiology, or disability, he was inspired simply as a humanitarian to strive to resolve the epidemic of ischemic ulcers and pressure sores among wheelchair users.

Graebe understood a bit about fluid dynamics, that both water and air dispersed among solid objects. It then struck him that if the body was supported on such a "fluid" surface, pressure would naturally distribute away from pressure points while surrounding tissue remained supported.

By 1973, Graebe incorporated his invention as "ROHO," the first complex rehab technology pressure management cushion. Unlike foam cushions, Graebe's design used joined air cells that were approximately four inches tall, and two inches in diameter. As an individual sat on the cushion, pressure points compressed the immediately underlying air cell, distributing pressure away from it.

Graebe, like his contemporaries, saw a need in the lives of those with severe physical disabilities, and rather than leaving all as idle observation, he acted upon his vision. Indeed, it's such pioneers as Graebe, who forewent the status quo, and set the complex rehab technology realm into motion.

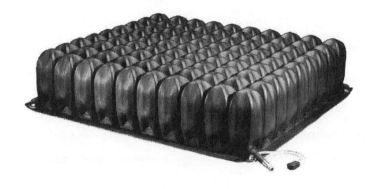

ROHO Cushion

Adding a Tilted Perspective to Complex Rehab Seating....

In the 1970s, wheelchair seating and pressure management products were static-based. While Graebe and subsequent manufacturers of pressure management cushions focused on the cushion and support aspects of seating, Greg Peek, a race car builder and driver who set a 235 mph record on the Bonneville Salt Flats, had a different idea.

In 1976, Peek was first exposed to wheelchairs while adapting buses for the Denver transit system.

"I was a fabricator, and had a contract to create a wheelchair securement system for the buses," recalls Peek. "I knew nothing about wheelchairs, so I went to really the only wheelchair shop in town and met Dick, a paraplegic who ran the place. Dick taught me what I needed to know, and I went to work on the bus project."

Peek and the local wheelchair provider remained friends, and in 1982, Peek was approached for a new project.

"Dick supplied Craig Hospital, and they wished a power recline system that put less stress on the bodies of quadriplegics as it reclined," shares Peek. "Dick gave me the job of creating it, with the only real instruction being to make sure that it worked with a ROHO High Profile. Driving home, I already had the idea of a high-pivot, low-sheer power recline in my head."

Peek's ultimate recline system worked, and he rapidly began conceptualizing and building "weight-shift technology," where those with a severe disability could have their weight shifted without being moved from a seated position.

"I worked with both recline and tilt, power and manual wheelchairs, and things caught on," recollects Peek. "We went to the first incarnation of Medtrade, with a ten-by-ten booth, not knowing what to expect. Our booth ended up being flooded with eager practitioners the whole show, and our newly-named company, LaBac, was a hit."

Peek's foremost concept was that by tilting the user's whole body rearward to 45 degrees at intervals during the day, pressure would be removed from the user's buttocks, dramatically reducing pressure sores. From Peek's tilt and recline systems onward, those with even the most severe of disabilities could perform life-changing weight shifts – an extraordinary advancement that we now know literally helps preserve lives.

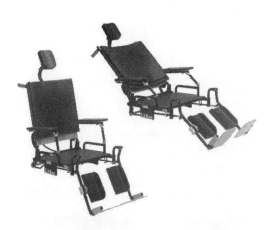

LaBac Seating System

In The First Person: Melissa's Story

I was 17 when my boyfriend, who, unbeknownst to me, had been drinking before he picked me up from my summer job at a Baskin-Robbins' ice-cream parlor. I didn't discover he was drunk until I woke up in the hospital weeks later from a coma, a C7-C8 quadriplegic.

I started rehab in a manual wheelchair that I could barely propel indoors – no way, outdoors. And, if that wasn't frustrating enough, my 90-pound, 5'6" figure was mostly skeleton, with pressure sores immediately putting me back in bed. It was devastating. I thought I'd have to spend the rest of my life in bed.

I now know I was lucky because it was the 1980s, and technology and wheelchair funding was there for people like me. My power chair with tilt seat and special cushion arrived, and for the first time in five months, I went outside. It was winter, but feeling the snow land on my nose was amazing.

My power chair not only gave me mobility, but prevented pressure sores. And, I could start rebuilding my life.

The Burgeoning Complex Rehab Technology Industry Gets put to the Test....

With complex rehab technology coming together – manual, power, and seating – it was increasingly evident that the ever-growing field was all but unregulated. In the 1960s, to address the expanding prosthetic need, the Veterans Administration established the Prosthetics Device Evaluation Center in Castle Point, New York, to ensure the quality of prosthetics. However, wheelchair technology was excluded and ungoverned. By the late 1970s, with complex rehab technology and the independent living movement gearing up, substandard complex rehab technology products were an increasing concern. For example, the most prescribed power wheelchair of the 1970s featured dangerously flimsy caster forks that consistently failed, stranding users. However, because there were no testing standards or governing compliance body, the manufacturer didn't address the issue.

In August of 1979, at the Interagency Conference on Rehabilitation, a formal organization was proposed, one that would create standards and practices to help regulate products and services within the complex rehab technology industry. Six members proposed the resolution, and 200 members immediately signed on, from engineers to academics to researchers to practitioners. Jim Reswick, Ph.D, was named the first president, his background dating to assistive technology advances in leg braces at Massachusetts Institute of Technology in the 1950s, and Robert Graebe of ROHO provided $1,000 in seed money. In 1980, the organization was formally established as a non-profit, under the acronym RESNA, representing its full name, Rehabilitation Engineering Society of North America.

RESNA worked throughout the 1980s to promote elevated standards within the complex rehab technology industry, formally publishing its first wheelchair standards in 1991, with the Veterans Administration and U.S. Food and Drug Administration both "recommending" that manufacturers adopt the standards. However, it would be another 14 years until the Centers for Medicare and Medicaid Services actually required that manufacturers meet RESNA standards in manufacturing wheelchairs.

As Rory Cooper, Ph.D., of the University of Pittsburgh, noted in a paper on wheelchair testing standards, "In this century, CMS, in what might be classified by some as an uncharacteristic move, has provided leadership in evidence-based classification of wheelchairs."

In the end, it was among the industry's founders who created testing standards that, while it took some time for formal implementation, dramatically raised the bar in providing complex rehab technology, all the way to include governmental regulatory requirements.

Reinventing the Power in Power Chairs....

With an added emphasis on standards and safety, as well as the evolution of power wheelchairs, batteries remained a questionable, outdated technology.

Power wheelchairs began as 12-volt systems, then moved to 24-volts, but the "deep-cycle" batteries never evolved. Up through the early 1980s, power wheelchair batteries were "unsealed, flooded" technology, meaning not only did they require monthly servicing with distilled water, but if tipped, acid poured out and, when charging, fumes filled the air.

Two gentlemen named Mark – Mark Kettler and Mark Wels – were golf cart and electric vehicle industry veterans who went into the battery business to service the golf cart and industrial vehicle market in Southern California (aptly named MK Battery after Kettler's initials). As they looked into what other markets might benefit from their battery business, they came across power wheelchairs.

"It just so happened that there was an Abby Medical store around the corner from us, and we inquired what type of batteries power chairs used," recalls Wels. "We learned that the whole mobility industry used flooded batteries, and immediately realized that flooded batteries were the least practical battery for power chairs, actually dangerous."

Dennis Sharpe, of Abbey Medical in the 1970s, and later to join MK, recalls, "Flooded batteries were especially dangerous for my pediatric clients. Pediatric power chairs were designed so unstable back then, and when one tipped over, battery acid spilled everywhere."

Kettler and Wels knew of a patented German battery technology that consisted of "gel" that didn't need maintenance and couldn't spill.

"Gel batteries seemed perfect for the wheelchair industry, but we had two problems," recalls Wels. "Firstly, no one made a 24-volt charger for gel technology. And, secondly, we'd have to convince the entire industry to accept a new technology if we were to succeed. But, it all seemed too meaningful to fail at."

Kettler and Wels secured the rights to the "gel" battery, worked with Lester Electrical to develop a charger, and then pounded the pavement to convince the complex rehab industry that it was a safer, more reliable technology.

"It was a tough sell in the early days, but by 1988, we had poured so much of our hearts and souls into getting MK batteries into one chair at a time, provider by provider, that we knew complex rehab had to be our mission," shares Wels. "We sold off the other parts of the business, and just focused on MK mobility."

Maintenance-free and safer, the MK Gel battery became the industry standard, supplying complex rehab consumers from coast to coast, where power chair safety and reliability dramatically increased.

"We struggled in those early years," says Kettler. "But, the complex rehab industry and consumers welcomed us into their fold. It was like a family, and we just wanted to help."

Breaking the Mold with Seating....

While ROHO focused on adapting its pressure management cushions to a range of those with disabilities, 1982 brought complex rehab seating to the next level of individualization.

Michael Silverman was shortly out of college when he hypothesized that the ultimate in positioning for those with severe disabilities, especially postural asymmetries, may not be adapting linear seating, but actually molding the seating to the client.

"My father was an orthotist, and I grew up working with him and those with disabilities," explains Silverman. "We provided support for the Muscular Dystrophy Clinic, in some cases creating orthotics for kids who were also full-time wheelchair users. When some of them came back to the clinic, I noticed that the orthosis weren't used, and when I dug in, I realized that they weren't being worn outside of clinic. They were just too hot or uncomfortable. Could we build the support into the wheelchair, so these users could get the support they needed without using an orthosis?"

With his father's encouragement, Silverman began working with Douglas Hobson, head seating researcher in the rehabilitation engineering lab at the University of Tennessee in Memphis. Hobson developed the MPI seating system, which in itself was a hard-shell seating "orthosis," primarily intended for use with children who had cerebral palsy and other conditions causing asymmetrical posture.

"The MPI system was great for its time," recalls Gerry Dickerson, an assistive technology professional who started in complex rehab in 1975. "However, parents were put off because there was no padding or such."

However, Silverman knew of liquid polyurethane foam and vacuum-formed vinyl, and pictured combing such soft materials with molded seating, tailoring it to each individual. One evening, at Elvis Presley's favorite bar in Memphis, one of Silverman's colleagues handed him the materials needed to make the first soft, molded seating system prototype.

Silverman's concept worked. By mapping one's body, and transferring that "silhouette" to his forming process, seating could be molded to the client, creating the ultimate in postural support and pressure management.

Still, what made Silverman's concept even more remarkable was that the mapping could be done at local providers, with Silverman transferring the data to his manufacturing process, delivering a one-off seating system virtually anywhere in the country.

In a rare opportunity, Silverman was allowed to demonstrate his product and process at the 1982 RESNA conference.

"There was dead silence in the room," recalls Dickerson. "Then we all realized that Silverman had revolutionized complex rehab forever by making truly custom seating a commercialized item. We stood in ovation knowing that someone had finally found a way to deliver a totally individualized product to us."

Silverman's newly formed company, PinDot (cleverly named after a fabric swatch that his mother had), along with pioneering practitioners like Adrienne Falk Bergen, began custom "forming" seating to individual clients. In particular, the Chicago Seating Institute was established, focused on PinDot technology, quickly growing from creating custom-molded seating for 15 clients the first year, to serving over 200 annually in the immediate years to come.

As Silverman wrote in a paper of the era, "…The most important thing a positioning system can do for the client is to aid in increasing his function, allowing him to continue with normal activities of daily life for as long as possible."

Indeed, Silverman's words could prove as the mission statement for complex rehab technology.

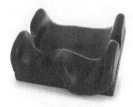

PinDot ContourU Custom Molded Cushion

Where Technology and Independence Met....

With complex rehab technology offerings expanding, those with severe physical disabilities pursued increasing independence and social inclusion.

The epicenter of the Independent Living Movement was Berkeley, California, where in 1972, Ed Roberts, a polio survivor relying on an iron lung, founded the first Center for Independent Living.

By the 1980s, the Independent Living Movement – which emphasized education, career, and societal equality (including universal access), for those with disabilities – spread nationwide. With the quest for independence came the need for more durable, adaptable mobility technology, and so as complex rehab technology improved, those with disabilities accessed greater independence and social inclusion, thereby needing even better technology. Put simply, technology allowed greater independence, and independence required greater technology, the two driving each other.

In the early 1980s, Berkeley remained the Mecca of the Independent Living Movement, where those with disabilities flocked to attend college, work, and secure accessible housing. In circa 1983, you couldn't stroll Berkeley's Ashby, Shattuck, or Telegraph Avenue without being amidst those using power wheelchairs. This integrated community allowed those with disabilities to lead the most independent lives, and many were frustrated by the lack of durability of commercially available power wheelchairs.

With such talent and motivation among those from the Center for Independent Living, U.C. Berkeley, and the community at large, a grassroots effort birthed what was known simply as the "Berkeley Power Chair." Without formal engineering or proprietary design – known in modern computer terms as "open source" – the Berkeley Power Chair featured a rudimentary welded rigid frame, chain drive, a used Porsche seat (for its pressure-management properties), and 12 inch go kart drive wheels. From there, many components from the user's existing power chair, including electronics, casters, and legrests, were incorporated. By commercial standards, it was a hodgepodge of parts, but it offered unmatched performance and durability, with even Ed Roberts using one with a ventilator on the back till his death in 1995.

No, the Berkeley Power Chair wasn't commercially available or attractive. However, it helped show the ever-growing complex rehab technology industry that those with disabilities needed increasingly-durable mobility products to live increasingly independent lives.

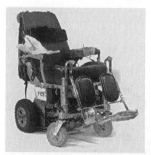

Ed Roberts' "Berkeley Power Chair"

Part Two
Complex Rehab, the Bold New World

The Sun Rises in Complex Rehab....

The mid 1980s ushered a flurry of activity in complex rehab technology, with products ranging from specialty drive controls to positioning products manufactured in garages and tiny shops across the country.

"It was a wild time," recalls Gerry Dickerson. "On the one hand, you had people like Whitmyer making awesome headrests that we used to have to make ourselves. But, on the other hand, people were just throwing contraptions at complex rehab to see what would stick. It was both an innovative and unorganized era."

Princeton graduate and business icon, Dick Chandler, saw both the innovation and chaos in the marketplace and wanted in, seeing tremendous opportunity in conglomeration of the complex rehab industry. After tenure in management at the Sara Lee Corporation, which owned Abby Medical, a leading national DME, an investment group bought Abby Medical in 1979, naming Chandler as president. By 1981, the group sold Abby Medical to American Hospital Supply, leaving Chandler to venture out on his own.

Chandler recognized that no single company dominated the manufacturing of a wide range of durable medical equipment, and surmised that if one could bring leading brands under a single company, exponential success was achievable. On January 18, 1983, with capitalization of $50,000, Chandler incorporated Sunrise Medical, Inc. with the goal of being the largest manufacturer of durable medical equipment and home health care products in the world. Within months, he raised another $5 million, and began acquisitions.

With several mobility manufacturers in his portfolio – A-BEC, Freedom Technologies, and Guardian – Chandler bought the widely-courted company, Motion Designs, home of Quickie, in December of 1986. Marilyn Hamilton, co-founder of Motion Designs, joined the corporate culture of Sunrise Medical as a vice president while her two partners chose retirement from the industry.

However, with the Motion Designs acquisition, Chandler was just getting started. Chandler saw the momentum both in Sunrise's portfolio growth and within the complex rehab market at large, and he wanted to dominate all sectors of complex rehab.

In an unconventional move, Chandler went to Japan, learning efficiency and corporate culture from such companies as Toyota and Matsushita, returning to the U.S. on an 18-month strategy to position Sunrise's operations and culture as mechanisms for success.

Chandler renamed Motion Designs "Quickie Designs," and established it as its own culture, with Sunrise's financial backing for growth. New practices and procedures were implemented, where production employees were encouraged to express better ways of manufacturing, and management had 72 hours to address it; and, call wait times for customers were reduced, decreasing the hang-up rate from 23 percent to 2 percent. Then, Chandler implemented a strategy that he learned in Japan called a "corporate growth conference," where he brought together Sunrise's division leaders to strategize faster growth. And, it worked.

By the late 1980s, the Quickie brand dominated the complex rehab market, with 1990 introducing its first power wheelchair. No other company offered the over one-million product variations that Quickie offered, resulting in a 50 percent market share.

With Quickie as its flagship brand, Sunrise Medical went from $140 million in revenue in 1998, to $319 million by 1993, named by *Forbes* as among the *Top 200 Emerging Growth Companies* along the way.

Indeed, Chandler accomplished his goal, demonstrating enormous potential in the conglomeration of complex rehab products, and it wasn't going unnoticed by the competition.

Technology and Equality Merge on Capitol Hill....

On July 26, 1990, President George H. W. Bush signed the *Americans with Disabilities Act* (ADA), into law, proving as essential civil rights protection for those with disabilities. The passing of the ADA was akin to the *Civil Rights Act of 1964* that made discrimination illegal if based on race, religion, sex, or national origin. For example, employers could no longer deny a qualified individual a job due to disability. Of course, the signing of the bill knocked down enormous social barriers, and those with disabilities could seek greater levels of social inclusion than previously known.

Interestingly, although the ADA was passed as civil rights legislation, it also recognized the requirements of complex rehab technology in the lives of those with disabilities. *Title III* of the ADA addresses public and commercial accommodations, specifically noting such aspects as dimensional space requirements in areas required to have wheelchair access, such as restrooms and buses. The standards were sanctioned by the American National Standards Institute, but set forth by RESNA, with such prominent figures as Sheldon R. Simon, M.D., an original RESNA founder, testifying at the Senate hearing for the ADA. Evan Kemp, Mal Mixon's friend and inspiration toward designing better complex rehab products, sat next to President Bush – in an Invacare power chair, no less – at the bill's signing.

With the signing of the ADA, those with disabilities had more social inclusion than ever before, and complex rehab technology and services were the tools needed to access the newly-granted rights.

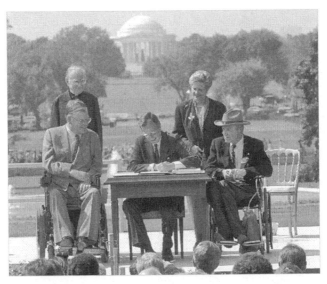

Signing of the ADA, July 26, 1990

In the First-Person: Julie's Story

Many people don't realize that where assistive technology and civil rights meet is where independence occurs. You can't have one without the other. I'm a child of the '60s, born with spina bifida, and have seen the tale of two cities – before mobility technology and the ADA, and after them.

The fact is, we needed wheelchairs that were the right kind in order to go to school and work. But, we also needed the legal, civil rights to do so. You can have a great job, but if you don't have the right wheelchair to get you through the day, you've lost the job. And, you can have a great wheelchair, but if you don't have legal rights toward transportation and employment, what's the point?

And, so, 1990 was a great year because both technology and civil rights for those with disabilities emerged and converged.

Complex Rehab Ricochets Across the Atlantic....

This book's preface rightfully states, "This book's intent isn't to overlook the global markets, but to focus specifically on the United States, where the lack of globalization and communication technologies of the 1970s and 1980s didn't allow the global exchanges that we have today toward products, practices, regulations, and services."

However, one company proved a dramatic exception, where a concept went from the United States to a rural town in Sweden, only to return 26 years later as state-of-the-art complex rehab technology.

In 1963, in the town of Timra, Sweden, Per Udden was a medical doctor and father of nine when a rehabilitation specialist from Los Angeles visited him. Dr. Udden, who had been forever troubled by the way those with disabilities were all but shunned by Swedish culture at the time, was inspired to learn about early power chair projects in the U.S. Dr. Udden saw power chairs as a way to liberate those with disabilities, and immediately went to work building a prototype in the basement of the medical center where he worked. His goal was to use such a mobility device to allow those with severe disabilities freedom from their homes, mobilizing them in the real world, increasing social inclusion and removing stigmas.

Dr. Udden built the first prototype himself, and in realizing its liberating qualities, joined forces with Countess Marianne Bernadotte, daughter-in-law of the King, creating political and

37

social awareness of supporting those with severe disabilities via mobility technology. By 1966, with remarkable support from Swedish officials, Dr. Udden, then working with several engineers, unveiled a pre-market prototype, unique with large front drive wheels especially intended for outdoors use. However, where Dr. Udden's design really acceded was in its seating – far ahead of its time – featuring power tilt and swing-away legrests.

Still, a name was needed, and Dr. Udden's wife suggested the obvious, combining Dr. Udden's first name with *mobil*: Permobil. As a further example of Dr. Udden's attention to social awareness, he created the logo in such a way that a slanted *e* represented a smile; the *o* represented a wheel; and, a disjointed *i* represented that no one is perfect. Yet, Dr. Udden took the Permobil brand as a social cause even further. In 1968, in Stockholm, he released an eight-minute avant-garde film showcasing celebrities and those with disabilities using the Permobil in the real world, from shopping to golfing. The film raised awareness for both Permobil and those with disabilities, dramatically improving social inclusion.

With the Permobil highly in demand by 1970 in Sweden, Dr. Udden took on an extraordinary manufacturing partner, SAAB, the car maker. Throughout the 1970s and 1980s, under Dr. Udden's leadership, the Permobil flourished in Europe, known for exceptional quality, while funding and disability support services evolved, as well. Dr. Udden, as proven, didn't just change mobility products; rather, he likewise changed for the better how those with disabilities were socially integrated.

By the mid 1980s, a New York-based distributor tried importing and selling the Permobil in the U.S., with little success due to non-translated literature, and a front-wheel-drive design that few recognized at the time. However, in 1989, Dr. Udden's son, Goran, came to the U.S., and "Americanized" the Permobil with U.S.-sought features.

The Permobil was slow to catch on in the U.S., namely due to its high price points. However, it slowly gained traction, becoming renown in the complex rehab community for its ergonomic power seating, branded *Corpus*. Unlike North American complex rehab seating systems that were very boxy, mechanical, and non-adjustable at the turn of that decade, the Corpus seat was ergonomic, sleek, and followed the silhouette of the user's body. In an era when the U.S. was evolving its form of complex rehab seating, Permobil jumped in with refinements from Sweden that few had fathomed developing.

"It was the power seating alone that led me to get a Permobil in 1992," shares Andrew Yarborough. "Their seating just was so much more refined than anything in the U.S. market."

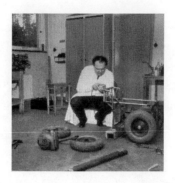

Dr. Udden's First Permobil Prototype

Complex Rehab Finds Its Own Home....

Up until the early 1990s, if one needed complex rehab technology, it was typically purchased through a durable medical equipment (DME) supplier referred by most in those days simply as a "wheelchair dealer." For consumers, it made getting the right technology difficult because most DME companies ran complex rehab technology as a sideline business, lacking professional expertise, and focused on commodity goods. However, Mike Ballard, a 42-year-old investment banker, by what he describes as an "act of God," saw exactly how the supply model for complex rehab technology needed to evolve.

"I was working on the finances for a DME when I found one segment of receivables that were much farther out than all other areas of the business," recalls Ballard. "When I asked about them, I was told to talk to the 'wheelchair lady.' She was just one woman, who seemed ignored by the rest of the company, and when I asked her about what she did, she showed me and I was immediately intrigued."

"The wheelchair lady" explained to Ballard how every wheelchair that she sold was custom to the individual client, and was a long, complicated transaction cycle, not like other areas of the DME business. Ballard then sat in on a client evaluation.

"There was a row of childcare's Quickie wheelchairs, and each was different. I'd never seen anything so diverse in DME," shares Ballard."Then a father brought in his three-year-old son, who had cerebral palsy, and when the boy got in one of the chairs and began pushing, his whole face lit up."

For Ballard, the experience resonated with his own life.

"My two boys were around three and four years old at the time, too, and it really touched me," recollects Ballard. "I still can't think of that moment of seeing the freedom that boy experienced without getting choked up."

Ballard immediately became passionate about complex rehab technology, and soon found himself pacing the aisle of the International Seating Symposium, the leading technology and educational conference for complex rehab technology practitioners and manufacturers.

"I was not only amazed at the products, but that there was a whole network of 'wheelchair ladies and gentleman,'" Ballard says with a chuckle. "But, the common theme was that they all were frustrated by the supply chain. They felt like a neglected part of DME, and it ultimately hurt clients because the big DMEs weren't prioritizing their needs. Someone in a rehab facility couldn't wait six months for a wheelchair, and that was par for the course in those days."

Ballard saw two areas needing change. Firstly, complex rehab technology as a business model needed elevated focus; it couldn't be a sideline business. Secondly, complex rehab needed to treat clients with true professionalism. Both the business model and social model toward delivering complex rehab technology had to change, and Ballard was ready to rise to the challenge.

"In 1992, I opened three National Seating and Mobility

(NSM) locations in the south," explains Ballard. "I hired the best rehab technologists that I could find. You had to have 10 years of experience, or you weren't on the NSM team. I then made each one like a 'doctor,' where I wanted them as the true practitioners among the staff. No sales people, no formularies, just true practitioners."

Being a self-proclaimed "computer guy," Ballard went to work automating the business.

"We couldn't have clients waiting six months for a wheelchair," says Ballard. "So, I wrote computer programs that expedited the processes needed to supply complex rehab technology. I remember rumors flying that we had some revolutionary 'code,' when really, I just set up NSM to run as efficiently as possible, knowing the importance of getting clients their needed mobility as quickly as possible. We've had tenacity and innovation, not magic."

Ballard's business rapidly grew, with rehab technology specialists wanting to get on board, finally having a business model to fit their professional needs, and the needs of the clients.

"Once we started growing, I held manufacturers to the highest standards," says Ballard. "We demanded quicker delivery and increased durability. I remember telling manufacturers, 'In three years, we'll be your biggest customer, so get with the program now.' I guess it was gutsy to name a tiny start-up in the south, 'National Seating and Mobility,' but ultimately the name proved true."

In the First-Person: Miguel's Story

I think I got my first power chair in 1978, and it was just kind of like, Here you go. *There was no evaluation or fitting or seating system. It was just a generic power chair delivered by a hospital supply store.*

In having cerebral palsy, I needed a lot of modifications to the chair. I needed a wedge seat and a one-piece foot board, and some other stuff. The hospital supply had no idea what to do, so my mom and dad made everything. A lot of it was trial and error because even we weren't sure how to meet my needs. We did this for my next power chair, too.

By my third power chair, it was the 1990s and so much had changed. The provider specialized in wheelchairs and did a real evaluation on me. He was a physical therapist and spent about three hours measuring, observing, noting, and asking me questions. He made a report that said what I needed. And, I really didn't know what to think of it all.

A month later, I went to get my new power chair and couldn't believe my eyes. It had everything I needed built-in. The therapist-provider even custom-molded a cushion to my body. It turned out to be the most comfortable, functional power chair I'd ever dreamed, and it literally changed my life. I ended up going back to college, getting a Bachelor's degree in social work and vocational rehabilitation. It's still amazing to me what a difference the right specialist can make in getting the right wheelchair.

Complex Rehab Evolves Locally....

"Complex rehab technology has always been local," explains Paul Bergantino, now President and CEO of Numotion, among the nation's largest providers. "And, when I started Connecticut Rehab, I rightfully only focused on my local area."

For Bergantino, he was born into meeting the needs of those with disabilities, with his father owning a Connecticut-based pharmacy and durable medical equipment supply for over 30 years.

"In the 1970s and '80s, I helped my dad's technicians work on wheelchairs after school," recalls Bergantino. "My dad also had close friends who used wheelchairs, so while I understood the importance of mobility technology, I also was very comfortable growing up around disability."

In the mid 1980s, Bergantino's father sold the pharmacy, and after college and a short stint in the accounting department of Yale University, Bergantino went back to work at his father's old pharmacy.

"Complex rehab was seen as a niche, sideline businesses in those days, but I saw tremendous potential to do things right," share's Bergantino. "The owners of the pharmacy let me handle the complex rehab side, but after a year and a half, I was frustrated with the way things were done, wanting to do it better. In 1990, I quit my job on a Friday and started Connecticut Rehab on Monday. It was a challenge in the beginning, as with starting most businesses. My brother, Toby, had a lot of industry knowledge, so he was a great source of support. But, it was ultimately persistence and just truly loving what I did that got me through those early years. If I were making pizzas or bicycles, I wouldn't have done it, but because of the clients I served, any challenges or sacrifices I had to make made it all worth it."

Around 1990, complex rehab providers were still small in numbers and very regional, as Bergantino saw every day.

"When I started, complex rehab was still lost within the big DMEs, receiving little attention, and providers dedicated solely to complex seating and mobility were few. I recall me in Connecticut, Gary Gilberti with Chesapeake Rehab in the mid-Atlantic area, Mike Ballard with NSM in the south, and others who were dedicated to this specialty market. And, all of us were evolving in our own ways," shares Bergantino. "My challenge was that being so local, with such a small consumer base, it gave me virtually no voice with funding sources. It was very trying to serve clients when payers didn't understand the vital role of this technology."

Bergantino worked hard through the 1990s as an independent, and believed more and more that in order to best advocate for consumers, he had to unite with others who were as passionate as him about complex rehab, and expand the complex rehab technology providership business model. In 1999, Bergantino's Connecticut Rehab was acquired by ATG Rehab, backed by a private equity group that held several other complex rehab technology providers, and methodically expanded into other regions of the country while keeping each acquisition local in its operations.

"Complex rehab was – and is still – local," explains Bergantino. "Based on everything from the evolution of products to climate, complex rehab technology preferences vary from region to region, and we've always kept our team members locally focused. The latest chapter was to create an industry leading company through combining ATG Rehab and United Seating and Mobility to form Numotion. Even though we've grown, we will continue using our resources and reach as an advocacy agent. No matter where you live, you should have the fullest access to liberating complex rehab technology. I entered complex rehab to serve others, and although the scale of our company has grown, my mission is truer than ever: to help every customer pursue independence."

A Storm Changes The Complex Rehab Power Chair....

By the early 1990s, Sunrise Medical dominated the complex rehab power chair market, with stylish, durable, customizable models, most notably the P200. The P200 featured programmable electronics, a compact footprint, and a seemingly indestructible nature. In form and function, as was commonly shared by Quickie engineers of the era, it was based on the Berkeley Power Chair concept, making P200 extremely popular among the most active users. However, it still featured static seating, unable to easily adapt to any number of complex rehab power positioning products.

Invacare watched Sunrise's power products consume the market, but also saw opportunity to evolve the complex rehab power base.

"It was in the late 1980s when it occurred to me that a complex rehab power base truly needed to be Play-Doh," explains industry veteran, Hymie Pogir, then a vice president with Invacare. "If practitioners had a power base they could mold to virtually any user's needs, they would have a tremendous tool.

By 1991, Pogir's team went to work on a pure complex rehab power base, where he notes, "We knew that it had to be adjustable and adaptable in every way, from seating to electronics. It couldn't just be one or two aspects; it had to be adaptable to each client in every way."

Invacare went through an extraordinary number of prototypes over the following year, discovering a power base design that was highly adaptable.

"You could adjust the wheelbase, making it longer or shorter," describes Pogir. "The seat mounts allowed adjustable center-of-gravity, and almost any seat could mount on it, especially power seating. But, at the heart of it all were the new Mark IV electronics – really the first software-based system – that tied everything together. Power base programming, seat functions, and specialty drive controls all interfaced. There was nothing close to our electronics on the market."

In 1994, Invacare launched the Storm Series, a more adaptable power base than the complex rehab market had ever seen. Rehab specialists and consumers immediately gravitated to the Storm Series, making it the complex rehab standard within seeming months.

"It did catch on quick," recalls Pogir. "But, no one knew that we intended to launch it sooner, but we wanted the Mark IV electronics to meet the new FDA EMI standards [initiated by RESNA], so we delayed the launch. But, once it hit the market, it took off."

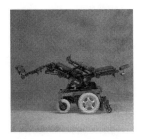

Invacare's Storm Series (Circa 1994)

Complex Rehab Technology Manufacturers Come of Age....

The Invacare Storm Series dominated complex rehab power bases in the mid 1990s, aided by several important acquisitions, including Canadian power seating manufacturer, Tarsys (an acronym for "tilt and recline system"), as well as Michael Silverman's PinDot line. Additionally, Invacare recognized the competitive edge that Dick Chandler brought to the market by offering a one-stop-shop for many complex rehab technologies, acquiring small manufactures ranging from the positioning components of Whitmyer to the seating surfaces of Jay Medical to the adaptive sports technology of Magic in Motion. However, Invacare wouldn't concede. Mixon, Pogir, and team wanted to be the one-stop-shop king, as well, in complex rehab, purchasing two small ultralight wheelchair manufacturers – Rowcycle and Top End – helping round their complex rehab technology offerings, creating its *Action* brand of products.

"It was an amazing time," recalls Gerry Dickerson. "As practitioners, we no longer had to farm-out components among small and big manufacturers. Finally, whether ordering from Sunrise or Invacare, we could get almost everything we needed in one order. It really served clients well."

The Power Chair Makes Another Turn....

By 1995, a third manufacturer was coming into the ring, but no one truly knew just what to make of it yet. Pride Health Care (now, Pride Mobility Products Corporation) was a leader in lift chairs (home recliners with an actuator that helped the elderly stand from the seated position), who went from lift chairs to manufacturing mobility scooters in the early 1990s. Scott Meuser, president, and his brother, Dan Meuser, vice president, realized that the same population that used lift chairs also could use mobility scooters, a logical market progression for the company.

In the mid 1990s, Pride was successful in the scooter market, with Dan Meuser focused on leading sales, and Scott Meuser focused on strategic planning. And, while Pride was presently working on a large outdoor scooter, a trip to Florida gave Scott Meuser a realization.

"There were power chairs, and then there were scooters, but nothing in-between," recalls Meuser. "I remember thinking that people needed something to get around their homes in. But, I wasn't sure what it should be."

Jim Mulhern, along with several other members of Pride's R&D team, headed up the project.

"We knew we needed something like a power chair, but more maneuverable indoors than what was on the market," shares Mulhern.

Traditional front- or rear-wheel-drive power chairs did well outdoors and were very stable, but required notable room indoors to turn. Mulhern and team wondered if a power chair could be made more maneuverable.

The team's ultimate concept was fairly simple in physics terms. If you wish to make a vehicle more maneuverable, move its drive wheel closer to center, so that it spins in a smaller radius like a top. And, that's just what the Pride team did. Whereas a front-wheel-drive power chair had the drive wheels and pivot point in the front, turning in a large arc (as with a rear-wheel-drive power chair), Pride's design shifted the front drive wheels closer to center, turning more on a mid axis.

"By moving the drive wheels toward the middle, the power chair turned in a smaller radius, and enhanced straight-line tracking," explains Jim Mulhern, named on the patents. "However, it made the power chair tipsy forward, so we had to address that."

Mulhern and his team mounted each side's drive wheel motor and wheel on a suspension pivot point and attached front anti-tip arms and wheels. Yet, simply adding forward anti-tip wheels didn't totally stabilize the power chair.

"I was driving a prototype and noticed that, based on the motor pivot point, the motor would raise and lower upon accel and decel," says Mulhern. "So, then, I thought, 'What if I attach the anti-tip arm to the motor?' And, it worked. When the power chair accelerated, the front anti-tip wheels lifted, and that helped with climbing obstacles. And, when the power chair decelerated, it pressed the anti-tip wheels into the ground, stabilizing the power chair. We really found something in that design."

Scott and Dan Meuser, not yet totally aware of the potential for Pride's "mid-wheel" design in the complex rehab market, wanted a name that applied to their known senior market – and the "Jazzy" was born.

The Meusers had a product that they knew would serve the elderly population well with its tremendous indoor maneuverability. Yet, others had their eye on the ingenuity of the Jazzy's design, as well.

"I knew there was something to that concept, the original Jazzy 1100 model, but just didn't totally get it at the time," recalls Invacare's complex rehab guru of the era, Hymie Pogir.

Pride opened the door to a new technology, but it would be several years before Pogir's and the complex rehab industry's questions were answered as to how the "mid-wheel" design fit in the complex rehab market.

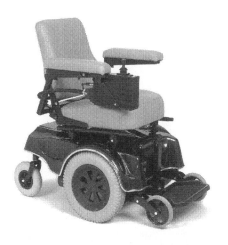

Original Jazzy 1100 (circa 1996)

Part Three
Complex Rehab, the Mainstream

Capturing the Nation's Attention Through Tragedy and Triumph....

On May 27, 1995, complex rehab made national news, filling the lead story on every network: *Actor Christopher Reeve is in critical condition this eve after a near-fatal equestrian accident....*

On June 1, 1995, Lois Romano, in the *Washington Post*, reported, "Actor Christopher Reeve, best known for his role as Superman, is paralyzed and cannot breathe without the help of a respirator after breaking his neck in a riding accident in Culpeper, Va., on Saturday. Reeve suffered fractures to the top two vertebrae, considered the most serious of cervical injuries, and also damaged his spinal cord, John A. Jane, the University of Virginia neurosurgeon treating Reeve in Charlottesville, revealed yesterday."

Reeve was stabilized and moved to Kessler Rehabilitation Center in New Jersey, with an ultimate prognosis of C1-C2 quadriplegia, among the most severe spinal cord injuries one can sustain. For Reeve, this meant full-body paralysis, including requiring a ventilator to breathe (although he eventually learned to breathe on his own for short periods).

During his time at Kessler, Reeve was prescribed a complex rehab power chair, complete with power seating for pressure management, sip-n-puff drive controls to use his mouth to drive the power chair, and a portable ventilator for breathing. As severe as his disability, Reeve knew the importance of complex rehab technology. In fact, among his first television appearances after his accident was on *Sesame Street*, where he demonstrated how he operated his sip-in-puff, as well as power tilt, noting to Big Bird, "With my wheelchair, I can do all kinds of stuff, including going to the library," and off he went with his son.

Reeve, arguably more than any other single individual, by nature of his openness and visibility, raised awareness to the importance of complex rehab technology and how it allowed him to pursue family, charity, travel, and, yes, acting and directing.

"That's like Christopher Reeve's wheelchair," strangers said to others using power chairs out and about.

No, the public didn't know the term, *complex rehab technology*. However, thanks to Reeve's heartfelt efforts in being such an advocate, many understood the vital role that complex rehab technology played in the lives of those with disabilities.

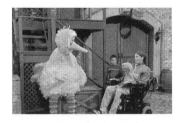

Christopher Reeve on *Sesame Street* (circa 2000)

And Then Complex Rehab hit the Web....

The late 1990s opened up complex rehab even further with a different type of technology: the Internet.

Up until wide-spread use of the Internet, many with disabilities lived segregated lives from one another, with no ability to share information. If an individual with a disability in Omaha needed complex rehab technology, his or her only source of information was a local provider and brochures. However, the Internet changed that isolation into a world of communication. With the Internet, one in Omaha could not only access information on complex rehab products, but also communicate with others around the country and globe. Whereas the Berkeley Power Chair literally never left Berkeley in the 1980s, suddenly those with disabilities were exchanging information at a rapid pace – that is, disability experience and complex rehab technology was no longer local, but global. In particular, niche complex rehab products now had a way to become visible to a much larger market, where companies like 21st Century Scientific (who aptly registered the domain, www.wheelchairs.com), and Permobil, the 1989 Swedish import still not widely-known by consumers at the time, began getting online buzz about their complex rehab power wheelchairs.

CurbCut.com was the first disability-related message board of merit, circa 1996, and when there was an overflow of discussion surrounding complex rehab technology by consumers, the need for a focused, consumer-based site was clear. This author started WheelchairJunkie.com in October 1996, and it immediately gained popularity among consumers and the industry.

"It was incredibly helpful to have a community to turn to," shares James Doty, a life-long wheelchair user and I.T. Specialist. "I finally had somewhere to turn for questions, answers, and input toward my mobility decisions."

Practitioners likewise used the Internet as a valuable tool to exchange information, from the RESNA Listserev A.T. Forum to RehabCentral.com. Soon, virtually all manufacturers had online presences, and the synergy of consumer, practitioner, and manufacturer interaction truly took complex rehab technology to heightened levels of shared knowledge, technology, and innovation.

In the First-Person: Hilton

There was very little choice in my neck of the woods in those days and one was entirely dependent upon the advice of dealers. WheelchairJunkie.com and the Internet at the time opened my eyes to a range of products, their pros and cons, and to how my disabled counterparts were using them to improve their daily lives.

Remember, there was no Google in those days, and, therefore, product reviews and experiences tended to be sourced from discussion forums. By the time I came to purchasing my second motorized wheelchair in 1998, I was able to make a far more informed decision, resulting in a product which provided a superior solution to my mobility requirements. More importantly, however, I saw how the motorized wheelchair could not only provide basic mobility, but also be a catalyst for change in my overall lifestyle. I was able to take on more responsibility within the workplace, which opened the opportunity for promotion and advancement within the company, a higher earning potential, and, therefore, a corresponding improvement in lifestyle. With financial independence came the security of owning my own home, motor vehicle, and the means to interact with the broader circle of friends and acquaintances.

Complex Rehab Technology Grows by One-Quarter Inch....

In 1996, David Lippes was a securities attorney living in Los Angeles when he came across a bankruptcy case that his firm was handling for a company called Sandvik. The roots of Sandvik dated back to the 1960s when two parent Swedish companies in the metals industry established Sandvik near Kennewick Washington. Sandvik served Boeing, and by 1984 began making titanium golf clubs under the brand, TiShaft, with its clubs ultimately winning PGA championships.

By the 1990s, Sandvik's Titanium Sports Division made bicycle and wheelchair frames, as well, including for Quickie. However, the sports market changed, with the golf club and bicycle businesses drying up, landing "TiSport" in Lippes' law office.

Lippes always wanted to run his own venture, and saw potential in resurrecting TiSport, purchasing it and heading to Washington. With Lippes at TiSport's helm in 1997, he quickly realized that the marketplace for titanium golf clubs and bicycle frames may never come back. Yet, he saw potential in complex rehab, ultralight wheelchairs. As the contract manufacturer for Quickie brand titanium frames, Lippes knew that Sunrise Medical understood the weight savings of titanium in ultralight manual wheelchairs, but they weren't truly innovating with the material. Sunrise Medical took its well-proven aluminum Quickie GPV model and simply converted it to titanium tubing. Lippes saw room for true innovation in design and split off from Sunrise

Medical, taking with him several wheelchair industry veterans.

Lippes sought to truly innovate in complex rehab ultralight manual wheelchairs, and he recognized that no one could make a better complex rehab ultralight manual than those who actually used them. He brought aboard industry veterans and users, Marty Ball as vice president of sales, and Alan Ludovici as vice president of engineering. For TiSport, it was the ideal marriage: Lippes had the management skills and technology, and Ball and Ludovici had intimate product and market knowledge.

By 1999, the three at the helm of TiSport rolled out their first model, the CrossSport. The market didn't just latch on to the CrossSport's efficient, durable, ultralight design, but to Lippes, Ball, and Ludovici's ideology that a complex rehab ultralight manual wheelchair truly is an orthotic device, an extension of the user's body, with a tailored fit to one-quarter of an inch. In fact, Lippes and Ludovici evolved a highly-computerized manufacturing process, where literally no two wheelchairs were alike, with each user's exact anatomical measurements transferred to engineering drawing, and a wheelchair then totally custom fit.

Soon, Lippes saw TiSport's line grow like wildfire in the marketplace. However, the name, interestingly, began holding it back, where insurers wouldn't fund "sports" wheelchairs, and it was at that point that TiSport became TiLite, adding not just a more funding-friendly name, but an ever-expanding line of totally custom-fit frame designs that helped ultralight manual wheelchair users lead the most independent, unencumbered lives possible.

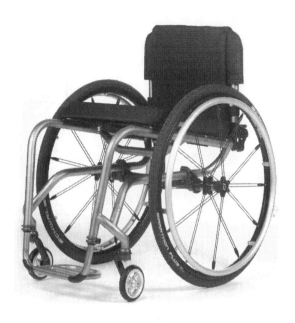

TiLite TR Complex Rehab Manual Wheelchair

Complex Rehab Technology Makes Quantum Leaps....

By the turn of the new century, 2000, Pride Mobility's Jazzy line captured notable market share in power chairs, with maneuverability being its hallmark. For the previous few years, beginning in 1997, rehab seating was slowly added as practitioners recognized the benefits of the Jazzy's tight-space handling and rearward stability for tilt seating. It was then that Scott Meuser of Pride Mobility recognized the potential and importance of focusing on complex rehab technology as its own platform, launching the Quantum Rehab division to innovate power bases and seating in this highly-specialized market segment.

"My brother Dan and I were excited about our big plan [to enter complex rehab] and we confided it to an industry leader. He said he liked the idea, but said, 'Don't call the products Jazzy. Don't even use Pride if you can help it,'" shares Meuser. "That's when we asked a creative member of our R&D group to come up with a name. We told him we wanted a name that reflected our desire to not be a 'me too,' but to be a force for propelling product innovation and value forward. He came back with one – Quantum. And with that, our new Quantum Rehab division was born."

"Quantum entered the market at an interesting time," notes Andrew Yarborough, lifelong complex rehab technology user and industry observer. "The major players were all seemingly trying to shift from the older technologies to truly advanced power base technologies, and struggling in that process to find a compass.

There were a lot of hit-and-miss products, and it hurt everyone. Quality was down, and there were some odd products being pitched that didn't meet complex rehab needs as well as they should."

Meanwhile, the Jazzy and Permobil increased competition in the market, arguably fueling the flurry of hit-and miss products that Yarborough witnessed.

"There was a lot going on, with new models being introduced to try to compete against Jazzy and Permobil," recalls Yarborough. Sunrise came out with a mid-wheel design that didn't match the Jazzy's performance, and Invacare had a less than perfect front-wheel drive that was nowhere near Permobil's evolved design. And, everyone expressed quality and service issues that weren't being heard."

During this turbulent time in complex rehab technology, as Yarborough points out, Meuser saw an opportunity to not just ramp into complex rehab power chairs with the newly-formed Quantum Rehab, but to truly make a difference in the marketplace.

"With the large volume of our Jazzy product line, we had developed tremendous power base manufacturing economies of scale. The next logical step was to use that scale toward the complex rehab power base marketplace," recalls Meuser. "Our goal was to use our scale and our R&D expertise to produce high-performance power bases and seating, and provide the rehab market with a premium product at a better value. At the time [2000], there was a widespread view that the economics of being a rehab provider were very unfavorable. We thought we could help change that. And looking back, I think we did."

"The Jazzy was a very successful product," explains Mike Ballard. "And, for Scott [Meuser] to roll that momentum into Quantum when he did was a very wise move that made everyone take note."

As Quantum Rehab began adding products to its line, others were acutely watching, including Hymie Pogir at Invacare.

"There was a lot going on during that time, with various 'mid-wheel' power chairs trying to compete against the Jazzy, then Quantum," recalls Pogir. "But, at Invacare, we were still married to the rear-wheel-drive. But, one experience opened my eyes. I was out visiting a disability advocacy group in Colorado when I encountered a little person perched way forward on one of our rear-wheel drives and her feet were dangling. I offered to send her free legrests, and she told me she had them, but couldn't maneuver in her home because her chair was too long. It was then that I realized that there was a real place for the mid-wheel power chair."

However, Pogir and his team at Invacare had their work cut out for them. Pride Mobility had patents locked up on mid-wheel technology. Plus, Pogir hoped to further apply complex rehab applications to the power base.

"I wanted to make a highly-maneuverable power chair that would conform to surfaces," shares Pogir. "Permobil had a chair in Europe for years that was six-wheel, with drive wheels in the center, so it was super maneuverable. But, it was more of an indoor chair. I remember telling my engineer on the way home from Colorado, 'We need something that's six-wheel, but can flex for uneven terrain.'"

At Medtrade 2003, Pogir's team demonstrated the TDX Series. Attendees gathered as Pogir's sales reps placed their toes against a wall, and rotated the power chair 360 degrees, ending up right back with their toes against the wall. By having front and rear casters for stability, and drive wheels truly centered, the TDX spun like a top. And, with suspension, the power chair climbed thresholds and conformed to uneven ground.

"I was impressed with what Invacare did with the TDX," says Meuser. "They truly took the complex rehab power base to the next level."

With practitioners and consumers driving innovation toward six-wheel technology, Quantum Rehab soon launched its Q6 Series, also featuring front and rear casters, with a center drive wheel.

"2005 was when Quantum really took off," recalls Quantum Vice President, Jay Brislin. "With our refined six-wheel power base and full power seating, we had the complete complex rehab packages that the market required."

With the TDX and Q6 lines in full effect, the market made six-wheel technology the new complex rehab standard. Six-wheel technology offered complex rehab power chair users extraordinary maneuverability, stability for power seating, and suspension for outdoor performance, making the most evolved, consumer-centric power mobility to date.

As noted by icons like Ballard and Pogir, Quantum's entrance and growth in the market inspired innovation in the industry, adding to the advancement of power complex rehab technology. For consumers and providers, expanded choice, performance, and value was a win-win for everyone.

"I remember watching the incredible innovations coming from Quantum and Invacare, and I thought, *Wow, the bar is being raised by the industry again. This is awesome to see,*" says Yarborough.

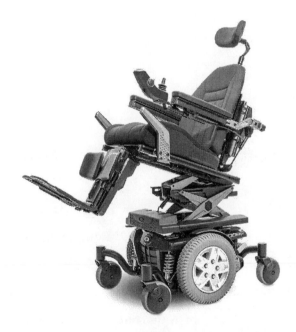

Quantum Q6 Edge with Full Complex Rehab Power Positioning Seating (Tilt, Recline, Elevating Foot Platform, Seat Lift)

In the First-Person: Tara

When you lose your ability to walk – in my case, due to multiple sclerosis – it's a strange experience. You go from the agility of a gymnast to driving a big rig through a shopping mall. At least that's what it felt like to me going from my own two legs to using a power chair.

And, my first power chair was a tank. 1 mean, it's hard enough emotionally trying to adapt to losing your ability to walk. But, then 1 was given this huge power chair, and maneuvering it in my small condo was worse than a bull in a china shop. 1 couldn't turn around in my bathroom, and 1 banged-up all my walls. The worst was when 1 knocked over a giant display of crackers at the grocery store.

My most recent power chair has the drive wheels in the middle, and 1 can turn on a dime. For the first time in years, 1 can turn around in my bathroom. And, it has an elevating seat, so 1 can reach my kitchen cupboards and the clothes hanging in my closet.

Even 1 didn't realize the difference that the right wheelchair can make in your life, and the maneuverability and functionality of today's power chairs make life so much more manageable and independent. So many things we take for granted, like just being able to turn around in your bathroom. When you can do it, then you can't, then you can again, it hits home how important mobility is.

Complex Rehab Technology as a Professional Practice....

The early 2000s marked a coming-of-age of the complex rehab technology providers – namely due to complex rehab practitioner and provider dedication toward creating industry standards for professionalism and continuing education.

In 1994, RESNA began evolving the Assistive Technology Supplier (ATS), and Assistive Technology Practitioner (ATP) certifications that were based on education, experience and testing. (By 2009, these two certifications were replaced by the single credential of Assistive Technology Professional [ATP]).

Similarly, during that time, the complex rehab suppliers – those who assess, fit, and provide complex rehab technology required to meet a person's identified medical and functional needs – formed the National Registry of Rehabilitation Technology Suppliers (NRRTS), specifically to recognize and regulate qualified individuals providing complex rehab technology.

Over the following decade, the two professional organizations evolved their standards and practices to ensure that only the most knowledgeable, ethical practitioners served consumers.

"There's no room in the complex rehab industry for anything less than the highest quality of practitioners," says Mike Ballard, founder of National Seating and Mobility. "Properly educated, experienced rehab technology specialists are true practitioners of care, and must be recognized as that."

Indeed, the ATP exam and NRRTS registration strive to

reflect the highest standard. When combined, a RESNA-certified ATP and NRRTS registrant must have rigorous educational and field experience, as well as meet standards of practice and continuing education credits. Additionally, a Code of Ethics is followed, as is available a formal client complaint process, punishable by revocation of certifications.

With RESNA and NRRTS working together, 2004 brought a third arm to protect and promote adequate coverage and access to complex rehab technology: a legislative advocacy body. Up until 2004, the American Association for Homecare (AAHomecare) represented the entire spectrum of home and durable medical equipment providers and featured the Rehab and Assistive Technology Council. However, rehab professionals felt that the organization's focus was so broad that it didn't have the ability to give complex rehab technology the legislative advocacy that it needed as a highly-specialized clinical practice.

"We greatly valued – and still do – what AAHomecare does," says Gary Gilberti, among the preeminent complex rehab technology providers and advocates, having started Chesapeake Rehabilitation Equipment in 1988. "However, those of us on the rehab council at the time felt like we needed a larger, more unified voice specifically toward complex rehab."

In a well-intended but somewhat controversial move, most members of AAHomecare's rehab council split off and formed the National Coalition for Assistive and Rehab Technology (NCART).

69

At the time, NCART co-founder and first President, Rita Hostak, vice president of government relations for Sunrise Medical, told *HME News*, "We are not trying to create two distinct worlds here. We still see AAHomecare as the voice of the industry on overall industry issues, but when you get to specifically high-end rehab and assistive technology, that's where our focus will be."

"We immediately went to work on that mission," says Gilberti, subsequent NCART president. "I mean, when you look at the re-coding [by the Centers for Medicare and Medicaid Services] of complex rehab products during the initial years of NCART, we, with NRRTS, spearheaded that fight. All who have supported our efforts continue helping us protect both access and quality of service for clients."

Part Four

CMS Intervention and Congressional Legislation

As Complex Rehab Technology Reaches New Heights,
the Ttide Turns....

Up until January 1, 2005, complex rehab technology funding was stable. With the ADA 15 years old, manufacturers testing products in the most stringent ways (to RESNA standards and FDA medical device protocols), and certified ATPs as providers, those with disabilities had more independence than ever before, with access to life-sustaining complex rehab technology leading the way. What's more, insurer funding was well established, where many needing a complex rehab power chair, for example, qualified under a single Medicare funding code, K0011. For approximately 2 million Americans with severe disabilities, the system was working.

In fact, the system wasn't just working, those with disabilities were thriving based on the culmination of three decades of advances in life-changing complex rehab technology. Power tilt and recline seating was highly evolved by manufacturers like Permobil and Motion Concepts, with profound health benefits toward pressure management. Power chair bases were highly-engineered by manufacturers like Quantum and Invacare, dramatically increasing durability a performance, allowing greater community access to education and employment. And, manual

71

wheelchairs by manufacturers like Sunrise Medical and TiLite were phenomenally ergonomic, compact, and lightweight, reducing fatigue and enhancing independence. In all, Complex rehab technology was available at life-changing levels that few had ever dreamed. If there was a true coming of age of complex rehab technology, it was here.

However, while the quality of complex rehab products, practitioners, and regulations dramatically improved over three decades, to circa 2005, costs always remained remarkably stable, with mobility product costs staying below consumer price index (CPI) growth. For example, in 2003, the average Medicare reimbursement rate for a power chair was $5,699, and it stayed there for 2004 despite a 2.1 percent increase in the CPI (which would place a power chair's cost at $5,818). This trend of complex rehab technology prices remaining below annual CPI growth during the previous decades proves remarkably consistent.

By all accounts those most in need of complex rehab technology were receiving the life-sustaining products and services requires, with levels of regulation and pricing that served all.

CMS Lays Down the Gauntlet....

Despite the first years of the 21st Century being a time of unparalleled liberation for those with disabilities, January 1, 2005, began a slippery slope for those most in need of complex rehab technology.

As the 108th Congress was seated two years earlier, it proceeded with the Federal Employees Health Benefits Plan (FEHBP), intended to revise Medicare services and include cost reductions (more commonly known as the Medicare Modernization Act of 2003). The Office of Inspector General (OIG) surveyed the market, and recommended that CMS reduce power chair funding by up to 20 percent. The OIG's argument was that, put simply, "free-market pricing" was below that of governmental reimbursement rates, a point greatly disputed by the industry and public officials alike.

In a May 13, 2004, letter leading up to the new year's FEHBP cuts, Rep. Bill Thomas (R-Calif), wrote, "During the rule-making to implement this provision, the Secretary should also evaluate whether there are significant clinical differences between the two populations - FEHBP and Medicare - which may affect the price of DME."

Indeed, what Rep. Thomas recognized was that beneficiaries needing power chair technology should not be categorized with those needing less-intensive benefits. The complex rehab technology industry's position was that the OIG's data was flawed, unrepresentative of true market conditions, including the levels of service needed to support mobility needs, not straight acquisition costs.

In representing the industry's view of the OIG report at the time, Cara Bachenheimer, Invacare's vice president of government affairs, said. "If I was CMS, I would be looking and thinking a little harder perhaps before just blindly implementing the reductions."

After a rally by the industry, with pressure on CMS by legislators, in late 2004, CMS agreed on a 3.28 percent reimbursement cut on power chairs, implemented January 1, 2005.

While the original FEHBP funding cut was a blow to beneficiaries, providers, and manufactures, there was another storm brewing that could potentially cut funding by at least 25 percent more. However, were beneficiaries and the industry ready for another fight to help preserve complex rehab technology from its greatest threat yet?

And Then CMS Changed the Rules....

On November 15, 2006, CMS changed the rules of access to complex rehab technology, dramatically inhibiting access for those most in need.

Up until that time only a handful of insurer codes – namely K0011 and K0014 in the complex rehab power chair area – dictated funding, with the specification for any single individual's mobility technology prescribed by a physician and clinician. However, in what CMS determined as a way to curb "over usage" of power chairs (a position that disability advocates noted as ridiculous since no one chooses to have a disability and use a complex rehab power chair), CMS completely revised its coding system, compiling 64 new codes and slashing funding by up to 27 percent.

Despite a 14-month complex rehab technology advocacy panel that educated CMS on power mobility technology, CMS instituted changes consisting of 64 new codes (that were likewise ultimately followed by state Medicaids and many private insurers) that devastated beneficiaries. Unfortunately, those complex rehab technology users striving to lead the most independent lives, working their way off of the system, bore the brunt of CMS' policy change. The industry-standard complex rehab power chair with a speed of 6 mph and a battery range of 16 miles (newly coded as a "Group 4" device), was deemed by CMS as no longer funded. For those with severe disabilities striving to pursue education, career, and community, this was a major blow, where CMS would no longer fund such vital access-to-the-community technology. To make matters worse, CMS emphasized its funding complex rehab technology for in-home use only. On the elimination of Group-4 complex rehab technology, CMS wrote, "Group 4 [power wheelchairs] (K0868-K0886) have added capabilities that are not needed for use in the home. Therefore, if these wheelchairs are provided they will be denied as not reasonable and necessary."

However, CMS didn't stop there. Complex rehab technology stakeholder advocacy groups, such as NCART and NRRTS, had to fight tirelessly to retain the next level down of complex rehab power chair funding, known as Group 3. By CMS' definition, a Group 3 power base had a speed of 4.5 mph and a battery range of 12 miles. These specifications were well below the liberating complex rehab technology that those most in need received during the previous 15 years.

With the elimination of Group 4 power chairs, and the low performance capabilities specified for Group 3 power chairs, CMS furthered its cuts in access and funding by including an additional policy revision. In a November 16, 2006, bulletin, CMS emphasized, "It is important to understand that because of the new coding and qualification system, coverage criteria for [power mobility devices] are based on a stepwise progression of medical necessity, otherwise known as <u>LEAST COSTLY ALTERNATITIVE</u>." This policy gave CMS the discretion, per claim, to "down code" beneficiaries from a Group 3 power chair to a Group 2 (non-complex rehab power chair), often in contrast to the physician's orders.

By January 1, 2007, exactly two years from the first 3.28 percent funding cut, CMS' coding revision slashed overall funding by an additional 27 percent, eliminated Group 4 complex rehab power chair funding, diminished Group 3 power chair performance, and gave itself the option to down code beneficiaries out of complex rehab technology.

Indeed, it was a challenging time for the complex rehab technology industry – but, most importantly, consumers.

In the First-Person: Jeffery

I was blessed that Vocational Rehabilitation was covering my tuition. I was in my junior year in college, studying psychology. I worked as a roofer for 20 years, and while mountain biking with my twin boys one Saturday, I went over the bars. I remember hitting the rocky trail and being alert, but not being able to move. I was a quad.

In rehab, in 1999, they set me up with an 8 mph power chair. It immediately became my legs. It took me everywhere and gave me independence. It was like the more I could do, the more I wanted to do. And, I really wanted to go to college and make something of myself. My power chair proved invaluable in not just everyday living, but getting to and around school.

In 2007, I went to replace it, wanting the same or a similar model, and was shocked to find out that it wouldn't be covered. My Medicare and Medicaid downgraded me to a smaller, slower, less range power chair. It seemed like insanity to me. I was doing more with my life, trying to get off of government assistance by going to college, and Medicare and Medicaid didn't want to recognize or support that. Instead, they told me I could only qualify for a power chair to use in my home. They wanted me to go backward in life.

It was then that I knew I had to get involved as a consumer-advocate with NCART and my elected officials to tell everyone how wrong the Medicare cuts were – and are – for complex rehab equipment. We can't live or be self-sufficient in every way without the right technology.

The Complex Rehab Technology Industry Rallies Behind Consumers....

With CMS' funding cuts of 2005 and 2006, along with the 64 new codes, and an emphasis on limited beneficiary access – including CMS restating the in-home-use-only policy, and reserving the right to down-code – complex rehab power chairs, as beneficiaries had known them, were unobtainable.

"We simply could no longer fund what a client truly needed," stresses Gerry Dickerson. "We literally couldn't replace a client's old chair with one of equal capabilities. We'd spent decades building life-changing technology and services, and funding cuts and policies were eroding access."

There was a trickle-down effect from CMS' actions: beneficiaries experienced dramatically-reduced funding, providers struggled to support clients, and manufacturers could no longer sell many of the life-sustaining technologies that they'd offered for years. For example, in 1998, Invacare innovated the gearless-brushless motor that throughout the early 2000s, offered consumers an ultra-durable, quiet, high-performing, straight-tracking motor. It was a great technology for complex rehab power chair users. However, because CMS declared the technology as residing in the no-longer-funded Group 4 class, the technology was virtually impossible to obtain.

Still, complex rehab manufacturers didn't give up considering the grim circumstances facing consumers. Manufacturers worked diligently and fast to release "funding-friendly" models, with Invacare, Permobil, Quantum Rehab, and Sunrise Medical all hoping to provide models and technology that fit funding constraints while preserving many of the features needed by consumers. Cost had to come out, and that meant eliminating certain features and performance. However, manufactures strove to the best of their ability to protect consumers' needs.

"Most manufacturers were in the same boat," says Hymie Pogir. "And, no one wanted to see consumers bear the brunt of the cuts and changes. It was like, 'Here we are, what can we do to make this right by those we serve?'"

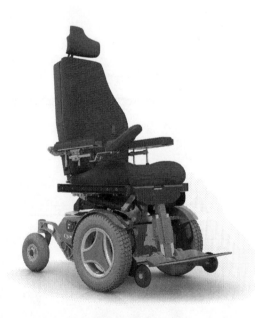

Permobil's C300 Corpus Complex Rehab Power Chair

Then, There's Competitive Bidding....

The term "competitive bidding" entered the complex rehab industry's lexicon in 2002 from other processes within the Medicare program. The core concept of CMS' Medicare competitive bidding of DME goods is that it divides the United States into 100 "competitive bidding areas" (CBAs), and requires DME providers to place bids to be one of the exclusive product supplier for Medicare in an area, and the lowest bidder wins. The concept sounded simple enough toward such commodity products as walkers or hospital beds. However, no two complex rehab products are alike, so the industry wondered how CMS could place a single funding amount on a product genre where no two units are alike.

In May 2004, newly-formed NCART immediately went to work striving to get complex rehab technology – and specifically Group 3 power chairs, which were included in the competitive bid program – exempt from competitive bidding.

"It was an easy point to make to CMS, but a tough battle to win," recalls Gary Gilberti. "It was really NCART's first big win for our consumers. And, it came from a lot of work by many complex rehab technology stakeholder groups."

The larger DME industry fought heart and soul against competitive bidding, believing it would diminish beneficiaries' access to quality products and services, and by 2009, several fronts were won. Firstly, Group 3 power chairs and accessories (the complex rehab technology included in Round 1) was permanently excluded by Congress from competitive bidding. This was a major win and significant sign that Congress was starting to understand the importance of complex rehab technology. Additionally, in exchange for a 9.5 percent funding cut on competitive bidding items and Group 3 power chairs, Congress delayed implementation of Round 1 in nine CBAs till 2011, and Round 2 in 91 more CBAs till July 1, 2013, taking the program nationwide.

Carving Out Complex Rehab Technology....

The funding battles that the mid 2000s brought for DME products and services put into perspective just how different complex rehab technology and services are from other product genres. Complex rehab technology (with the exception of the exemption from competitive bidding) has remained in the DME funding category, treated at times by CMS as a standardized item, although it's dramatically different. As a result, whenever funding or policy changes have been made toward DME goods and services, complex rehab technology has been negatively effected, sometimes directly, other times, indirectly.

NCART, NRRTS, and the complex rehab technology industry as a whole have striven since 2004 to have complex rehab technology recognized by CMS as its own benefits category, separate from DME, specifically due to the highly-individualized, prosthetic-like nature of the technology, where each unit is custom fit per individual. In fact, prosthetics-type classification is exactly where complex rehab technology belongs – that is, outside of the generalized DME product category.

"If you look at the fact that, by CMS' own policies, complex rehab technology must be prescribed and fitted by specifically-certified individuals, products are custom made for each individual, and the diagnosis warrants the prescription, it's clear that complex rehab technology and related services is closer to a prosthesis than any other medical device," says Paul

Komishock, general manager of government affairs for Quantum Rehab. "Therefore, it should have its own benefits category."

Interestingly, in seeking complex rehab technology as its own benefits category, no one wishes to increase funding. Rather, carving out complex rehab technology as its own separate benefits category would protect the technology – and, ultimately, beneficiaries – from further funding cuts within the general DME category.

The good news is that progress is being made within Congress to create a separate benefit category under the Medicare program similar to that for Orthotics and Prostehtics. In 2013 House and Senate legislation was introduced via the *Ensuring Access to Quality Complex Rehabilitation Technology Act.* The legislation creates a separate benefit category for complex rehab technology within the Medicare program, so that adequate access to these critical products and supporting services can be assured. The legislation appropriately distinguishes these specialized products and makes other required changes, including increasing related standards and safeguards, to better address the unique needs of individuals with disabilities and medical conditions who rely on complex rehab technology to meet their medical needs and maximize their functionality and independence.

Getting legislation introduced was the culmination of a three-year process, and it is only the first move. Thankfully, there is a large group of complex rehab stakeholder individuals and organizations from across the country that are hard at work getting additional Members of Congress to sign on as cosponsors to the legislation. This group of advocates includes consumers, practitioners, providers, manufacturers, and others committed to protecting access to complex rehab technology. The initial objective is to get Congress to pass legislation to establish separate recognition for complex rehab technology within the Medicare program, providing needed safeguards and coverage changes. From there, the policies and safeguards can be adopted by state Medicaid programs and private insurance plans. The success of this initiative has broad and positive implications toward protecting access to complex rehab technology products and supporting services. It's overdue and much needed.

Complex Rehab Technology Goes Back to the Future....

Despite funding challenges, the heart and soul of complex rehab technology is stronger than ever, with innovation occurring today in the same spirit of those who pioneered the field four decades ago.

"With so much technology in the world today, much of it yet to be integrated into complex rehab products, we've only scratched the surface," says Scott Meuser. "We're all in this for the long run of bettering the lives of our consumers, and it's all driven by product innovation. None of us even knew what Bluetooth technology was 10 years ago, but now it's built into power chair hand controls, where you can use the joystick to control a cell phone. I see everything from electronics to seating getting better and better from here."

Mal Mixon agrees, noting, "Those with disabilities want to live the fullest lives possible, and that only comes from knowing that everything can be improved, then doing it. We've all seen that the better the complex rehab technology, the more independence people have. So, we just keep building upon it."

"A lot of it is in just sticking to our mission," says Mark Wels. "In the evolution of complex rehab technology, we'll never stop pushing forward. This is about supporting our family and friends who have disabilities. The greater the technology for those with disabilities, the better our society."

And, Paul Bergantino sees tremendous potential toward progressing from a health care viewpoint, sharing, "Complex rehab technology is so much more than simply durable medical goods. I'm optimistic that we're heading toward a day when complex rehab technology will be rightfully seen by all as the encompassing health care solution that it is."

Indeed, the countless individuals passionate about complex rehab technology continue pushing the limits in an interest to improve lives. A host of next-generation pressure-management cushions are in development, some automated to circulate air through the cushion, deflating portions to reduce pressure points. Manual wheelchair "power-assist" devices get more advanced, where a push of the hand rims initiates a power boost from a "smart" power add-on device. And, power chair electronics interface more and more with the world we live in, having built-in environmental controls that can operate cell phones and home appliances, all through the hand control. These few areas of innovations and many more not only improve the health and independence of those with severe disabilities, but exponentially increase quality of life.

In the exciting present and future of complex rehab technology, consumers are, of course, the focus, and as James Doty points out, "From suspension to the color LCD hand control screen with all of the power chair's functions monitored at once like a car's dashboard, I never thought I'd see so much technology in one power chair. It's really fascinating for lifetime users like me to not just see how far complex rehab technology has come, but where it's going. It's changed my life, and I can't wait to see what it offers future generations."

Afterword

Complex Rehab Technology: The Great Liberator

As I've spent my own life as a beneficiary of complex rehab technology – it allowing me to blaze a path in mainstream education, attend college, earn a living, raise my daughter, and contribute to society – I've preached the gospel, one might say, as to the benefits of allowing my peers with complex rehab needs to have the right mobility technology to liberate their lives, as well.

In my many years advocating on Capitol Hill to everyone who will listen – senators, congressmen, the President – my message never waivers. See, when we, as a society, ensure that those most in need have access to life-sustaining complex rehab technology, everyone wins. Provide an individual who has a severe disability the appropriate complex rehab technology, and he or she can rightfully pursue education, career, family, and community. I can't count how many times I've witnessed an individual struggle to obtain the right complex rehab technology due to insurer bureaucracy or funding constraints, but once secured, he or she tackled education and employment with remarkable achievement, from being on the system to paying into the system. Wouldn't it be amazing if all with severe disabilities had such opportunity?

Yet, beyond any one individual's success, there are fiscal incentives for insurers to fund the appropriate complex rehab technology that benefit all. Obviously there's a direct, positive fiscal correlation in supporting an individual's shift from

89

beneficiary to tax payer by supplying the appropriate mobility to make him or her mobile toward pursuing activities of daily living. However, complex rehab technology is a proven tool in preventative health care costs. Complex rehab pressure-management cushions are a great example. Medicare spends $1 billion per year treating pressure sores, with the average patient treatment per sore costing $70,000 (not including the average six months required to heal, taking a socio-economic toll on the family and employment). However, it's estimated that a $400 pressure-management cushion can reduce the risk of pressure sores by 80 percent. Per individual, the numbers show a logical and real fiscal and health-based return on investment: spend $400 on a pressure-management cushion, and save $70,000, while also preserving the individual's quality of life.

Yet, Medicare and most insurers don't practice this logical, humane, fiscally-sound model. The predominant factor in determining if an individual qualifies through Medicare for a pressure-management cushion is a history of pressure sores. Literally, rather than recognizing that every complex rehab technology user is at risk for pressure sores (our buttocks simply weren't intended to support our weight indefinitely), and funding a preventative cushion, the agency will often deny the claim, then spend $70,000 on treatment when a sore develops – and, then invest $400 on a pressure-management cushion.

My point is, as a society, in order to rightfully extend full, productive inclusion of those with severe disabilities, complex rehab technology is the great liberator. Providing access to the right complex rehab technology allows preservation of health, rightful quality of life, integration within society, and optimal independence. When combined, it's clear the complex rehab technology has a profoundly important role in society: Equality for all.

Mark E. Smith
Pennsylvania
September 2013

About the Author

When Mark E. Smith was born with severe cerebral palsy, the doctors said that he was an absolute vegetable, void of cognitive skills. On top of that, Mark's family was fragmented by alcoholism, divorce, incarceration, and suicide. But, Mark simply defied all odds, turning facing the insurmountable into accomplishing the impossible – transforming his life from the trials of a severely disabled child with little to the triumphs of an adult fulfilling his dreams, including obtaining a master's degree.

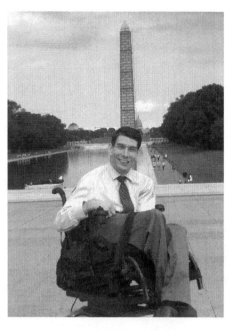

Today, Mark is among the most recognized disability figures in the world. His accomplishments are unmistakable as an icon within the complex rehab industry as a technology specialist, columnist, and consumer advocate. Mark is the author of four books and countless magazine articles and columns, is the Founding Editor of WheelchairJunkie.com, a leading website for those with disabilities and their complex rehab technology needs. And, Mark is a lecturer and sought-after inspirational speaker. Of course, Mark's most important role is that of father, raising his teen daughter, a nationally recognized youth scholar and musician.

See, when Mark speaks of shifting one's life from merely surviving to truly *thriving*, he doesn't just talk about it – he's lived it.

For more information, please visit www.wheelchairjunkie.com.

Made in the USA
Charleston, SC
27 January 2014